The Beginner's Guide to the Protein Diet

Effective Weight Loss That Works

By: Florence Perkins

I0439501

TABLE OF CONTENTS

Florence Perkins
PUBLISHERS NOTES

Disclaimer

This publication is intended to provide helpful and informative material. It is not intended to diagnose, treat, cure, or prevent any health problem or condition, nor is intended to replace the advice of a physician. No action should be taken solely on the contents of this book. Always consult your physician or qualified health-care professional on any matters regarding your health and before adopting any suggestions in this book or drawing inferences from it.

The author and publisher specifically disclaim all responsibility for any liability, loss or risk, personal or otherwise, which is incurred as a consequence, directly or indirectly, from the use or application of any contents of this book.

Any and all product names referenced within this book are the trademarks of their respective owners. None of these owners have sponsored, authorized, endorsed, or approved this book.

Always read all information provided by the manufacturers' product labels before using their products. The author and publisher are not responsible for claims made by manufacturers.

© **2013**

Manufactured in the United States of America

DEDICATION

This book is dedicated to my parents, who allow me to try new things.

CHAPTER 1- WHAT IS THE PROTEIN DIET?

The protein diet is incredibly popular because of its effectiveness at helping people lose weight fairly quickly. In this diet you increase the amount of protein you consume each day. For your diet to be considered high in protein it should be at least half protein but there are many variations available. Some of the most famous protein diets will restrict the amount of carbohydrates you consume while at the same time encouraging the consumption of protein. Others, however, simply recommend increasing the amount of protein you have each day and allow you to choose what foods you will cut out of your diet to make that goal.

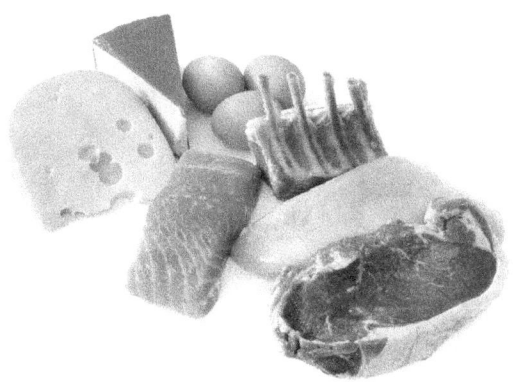

How It Works

Protein diets are effective because of several things. One of the main reasons is that proteins cause your body to increase the release of ketones into the bloodstream. These ketones lower your appetite so you aren't hungry as frequently. In addition, protein helps you stay full for much longer, reducing snacking throughout the course of the day. The forms of the protein diet that eliminate or reduce your intake of carbohydrates have the additional benefit of leading to fluid loss, helping you lose weight quickly.

Who Should Consider It

Experts say that everyone who is trying to maintain their weight or lose a few pounds should consider increasing their consumption of protein. Ideally though it shouldn't be used on a long-term basis as a protein diet isn't usually nutritionally balanced. Despite this, someone looking to give their diet a kick start would be a great candidate, especially if they are extremely overweight. It is a great way to help them control their hunger. High protein diets are extremely popular among bodybuilders as the increased protein helps you build muscle more quickly. Having protein after a workout also helps your body recover more quickly which is another reason why athletes with intense training regimes consider this type of diet.

Expert Opinions

In general, medical experts encourage the protein diet as a great option but most caution that you shouldn't do it for more than six months or so, although a slight increase in your consumption of protein can be done in the long term. They also point out that if you choose to increase your protein intake in general you need to be careful about what foods you choose. Instead of going with fatty meats, you should choose lean protein.

Considerations to Stay Safe

If the version of the protein diet that you are following involves a decrease in carbohydrates, you need to make sure that you don't stay on it for more than six months or so. That is because consuming fewer carbohydrates may lead to not getting enough fiber; therefore you should always opt for carbs that contain high amounts of fiber.

You should also avoid eating too much red meat or dairy products that are full-fat as this could increase your risk of developing heart disease. Another reason to avoid consuming extremely large amounts of protein for too long is that it can increase your risk of osteoporosis and damage some of your internal organs. If you take those concerns in mind, however, and limit the length of any diet that has a large portion of your calories coming from protein, you should see results and be completely safe.

How Much Protein

Although a high protein diet is generally considered anything with more than 50% of the calories coming from protein, you don't really need that much (which is part of the reason this diet is ideal to help you meet a short term weight loss goal or kick start your weight loss). Most experts recommend that you should have somewhere between 10 and 35% of your calories from protein each day. The recommended daily allowance is only 56 grams for men and 46 for women but if you want to stick to the protein diet, you should be aiming for about 120 grams.

Sources of Protein

If you plan on following the protein diet, then it is essential that you know which foods are excellent sources of protein. The following list shows not only the foods with the most protein but also the amount (in grams) found in a 100 gram portion of the given food item.

- Turkey breast (30 grams)
- Chicken breast (30 grams)
- Fish such as halibut, tuna or salmon (26 grams)

- Low-fat mozzarella cheese (32 grams)
- Cottage cheese (32 grams)
- Pork loin in the form of chops (25 grams)
- Lean beef (36 grams)
- Low fat veal (36 grams)
- Tofu (7 grams; despite this seemingly low number it has an excellent ratio of protein to calories with 1 gram of protein for every 7.4 calories)
- Mature soy beans (17 grams)
- Eggs (13 grams)
- Yogurt (6 grams)
- Milk (6 grams)
- Soy milk (6 grams)
- Nuts and seeds (33 grams; it is important to remember, however, that these have a higher protein to calorie ratio than some other items at 1:15.8 and can also be fatty)

When choosing your protein diet plan, you should try to opt for one that includes at least some carbohydrates. When selecting the carbs to eat, always go with ones that are healthier and provide you with plenty of nutrients such as fruits, vegetables and whole grains.

Tips to Increase Protein Consumption

Despite knowing which foods are rich in protein, many people have problems adding lean protein to their diets. Here are some ideas to help you easily add protein without much effort.

- When looking for meat, opt for tenderloin or round cuts.
- If you are looking for a snack, try edamame beans, hard-boiled eggs or fat-free mozzarella cheese, all of which are healthy and high in protein.

- If you want a breakfast option that isn't just eggs, try some lean sausages or smoked salmon.
- If you eat a bowl of cereal in the morning, add an entire cup of milk for the extra protein.
- If you prefer oatmeal in the morning, always make it with milk not water. This will not only add protein, but flavor as well.
- When you go to the gym, try taking a bit of yogurt with you. This is a great post-workout snack to help you replenish your proteins.

CHAPTER 2- WHAT ARE THE ADVANTAGES OF THE PROTEIN DIET?

Diets have been around for centuries. People use diets in order to lose unwanted weight so they can fit into a special dress, impress someone, or to become healthier. Through the years hundreds of diets have appeared but people may find that these diets are complicated, take too long to work, or they simply do not work at all. Individuals become disappointed and discouraged and may decide to end their attempt to lose weight. A protein diet has many advantages and can aid a person that is trying to lose weight.

No Special Foods to Buy

During a protein diet there are no special foods to buy. Some diets require that you purchase foods directly from them. In a high-protein diet you can just simply increase your intake of protein each day. The average American consumes 12% to 18% of their calories from proteins. Transferring to a protein diet will require one to increase this daily percentage.

For some, the protein diet requires that about half of their calories be from protein. This means that you get to consume more of the foods that you love to eat such as eggs, cheese, and meat. No need to consume foods that lack flavor, are hard to chew, are hard to find. With a high protein diet you are able to visit your local market to purchase the foods you need for this diet.

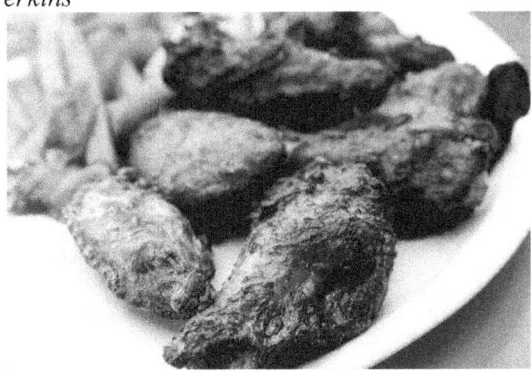

The Pounds Drop Quickly

A protein diet involves removing carbohydrates from your menu. When Carbohydrates are missing from your diet your body begins to burn its own fat for energy. This process is called ketosis. This means that every calorie that is burned will result in a calorie lost. Individuals will find pounds quickly falling off of them, as a high-protein diet helps to turn their body into a highly effective calorie burning machine.

Another reason why people on a high-protein diet lose weight quicker is because of their metabolism. Consuming high protein meals can help to boost your metabolism. Your metabolism is the rate to which your calories are burned. If you have an increased metabolism, this means that your calories will burn faster; calories that burn faster will result in pounds being eliminated quicker.

The result of a high-protein diet will be a weight loss of 4 to 6 pounds per week. This will allow a person to swiftly fit into an old dress or a newly purchased outfit. A regular diet yields a weigh loss of 1 to 2 pounds per week. With this comparison, high-protein dieters are able to help a person lose about 50% to 150% more weight than individuals that try other diets. This is great news because as individuals begin to notice how much weight they have lost, they will more than likely be inspired to continue on their diet until their goal is met.

You Feel Full

During a protein diet, your appetite is decreased because you feel full. This is a benefit for dieter because they do not have an urge to continue eating. One of the reasons for unwanted weight gain is the over consumption of certain foods. The body will reduce its need for unhealthy foods such as cookies, cakes, and candies because you will feel satisfied by the high-protein meal.

Other diets can leave you with an overwhelming feeling of hunger and a growling stomach. When this occurs, your mind can become consumed by the feeling of hunger and the result is you over indulging in high calorie foods that are not a part of your diet. This type of binge eating can cause you to regain the weight that you have lost and then more. Gaining more weight than you have lost can lead to discouragement and giving up on the weight-loss journey.

The Blood Can Become Stabilized

Individuals that are diabetics can find that a high-protein diet can cause their blood to become stabilized. This is because a person's blood sugar can become unstable when a person consumes a sugar. Consuming a high-protein diet can eliminate a lot of the foods that causes a diabetics blood to fluctuate. Carbohydrates and sugars will be consumed in less quantities resulting in a constant level of blood sugar. It is true that the body converts protein in to glucose, which is a sugar. But this conversion happens at a slow rate and will more than likely not have a vast effect on a diabetic's blood sugar.

Fight Diseases

A high protein diet can help to build muscle, make bones stronger, and maintain healthy cells. All of these benefits can lead to a healthier immune system. A healthily immune system can fight off certain viruses and diseases that can cause a person to get sick. If a person does get sick, the nutrients received through the diet shorten the amount of time a person is sick.

Producer of Lean Muscles

Athletes, body builders, or intense exercisers turn to a high-protein diet in order to develop lean muscles. A lean muscle does not include fat. A person that has a high amount of lean muscle has the appearance of having strength. This is true for bodybuilders, a high-protein diet is able to increase the size of their muscle and help them to win various contests.

Beyond aiding in the appearance of being strong, lean muscles help to increase one's strength. A high-protein diet can increase the amount of physical tasks can be performed by an individual. For an athlete or intense exerciser this is important because a high-protein diet is able to increase the amount of time they spending doing physical activity. The result can be a satisfactory workout or game.

The advantages of a high-protein diet are many. Whether a person is trying to fit into an outfit or prepare for a game; a high-protein diet can help them to reach their goals. Beyond having benefits to a person's image, a high-protein diet can be used to stabilize one's blood sugar or even assist in maintaining a healthy immune system. Whatever the reason for trying a high-protein diet, dieters will not be disappointed with the results.

CHAPTER 3- WHAT ARE THE MOST POPULAR TYPES OF PROTEIN DIETS CURRENTLY AVAILABLE?

There are several popular protein based diets that are currently available. These types of diets are very popular among dieters who want to lose weight, especially those who want to lose it fast. While some may be harder to maintain than others because of their restrictions, any high-protein diet should be followed with caution to avoid potential health risks and should not be used in exchange for an exercise plan, which is the most healthy and effective way to lose weight and manage it better.

The Zone Diet

Created in the 1990's, Dr. Barry Sears created a diet that would put dieters in the "zone" if their diet consisted of 40% carbohydrates, 30% protein and the same 30% of fat. The zone diet doesn't restrict that many food products as long as specified proportions for each meal are met, however there is a limit on how much bread, pasta and other certain foods that a dieter must follow on this diet. On this diet, dieters are encouraged to eat low-calorie meals on a regular daily basis to promote weight loss.

The South Beach Diet

The South Beach diet is one of the most healthiest high-protein diets currently on the market because it promotes its followers to consume whole grains, beans, legumes, vegetables, and low-fat dairy products in addition to the healthy unsaturated fats that's in olive oil, fish and nuts to encourage healthier eating habits in some ways.

However, this diet, which was founded by Dr. Arthur Agatston in 2003, is highly restrictive of other healthy foods such as fruits and carrots; Since the South Beach diet is based on the glycemic index, which levels food based on how long it takes their sugar to enter the bloodstream, fruits and carrots make it high on the index. The higher a food product is on the index, the more it should be avoided. This protein diet allows up to 20 to 90 g of carbohydrates for every meal.

The Protein Power Diet

This diet is 26% protein, 16% carbohydrates, 54% fat, and 4% alcohol. The Protein Power Diet, which was made by Dr. Michael and Mary Eades in 1996, is a bit similar to the South beach diet in the way that both diets restrict the intake of fruit. Starchy vegetables, grains, and milk is also restricted on the Protein Power Diet. However, this diet allows the consumption of non-starchy vegetables, butter, oil, meat, fish, poultry, salad dressing, eggs, and cheese.

Alcohol can also be consumed in moderation on this diet. The Protein Power Diet is very simple to follow while the carb counting may be the only downside; dieters are required to count the carbohydrates in everything they eat. A carb crash is also possible during the first week of this diet; carb crash is when the dieter feels fatigue and irritability when a new low carb diet is started and can last for several days while the body adjusts to the program. That can be said for the Power Protein diet, as well as any other high-protein diets that have low-carb consumption as part of their plans. While the effects of the 'crash' usually subside by the second week on the diet, the symptoms can be helped by eating half an apple or some vegetables to help ease your body through the transition.

The Stillman Diet

Out of all the high-protein diets that are currently available on the market, the Stillman system is the highest with 64% of protein, 33% of fat and only 3% of carbohydrates. Recommended guidelines for diets suggest that protein range from 10 to 15%, carbohydrates range from 40 to 60%, and that fat range from 20 to 35%, making the Stillman diet not meet these guidelines.

The reason consumption for carbohydrates is so low is because this diet was structured around the belief that carbohydrates store fat in your body while protein helps to burn fat. This diet restricts that consumption of carbohydrates such as bread, pasta, dairy products, fruit, and vegetables while also limiting fat and oil. Lean meat, poultry (without the skin), fish and seafood, eggs, and low-fat cheese is promoted as the only foods that should be eaten on this diet.

The Sugar Busters Diet

The Sugar Busters Diet has the highest intake of carbohydrates at 52% while protein only makes up for 26% and fat at 21%. This diet allows the consumption of all proteins, fats, and foods that are lowly leveled on the glycemic chart (Much like the South Beach diet.) while also allowing the moderation intake of alcohol like the Protein Power diet.

White flour (Food that is refined from it), white rice, bread, and potatoes are restricted on this diet, as are carrots, beets, corn, and carrots. Cake, cookies, muffins, pretzels, and other white flour products are forbidden. Canned fruit, and any product that contains added sugar, should also be avoided. Pasta that's whole grain can be consumed and bananas are okay as long as they're ripe and green. With this diet, it's important to note that wheat flour or not whole grain. Only whole wheat will be whole grain.

The Atkins Diet

Florence Perkins

The Atkins diet consists of 27% protein, 68% fat, and only 5% of carbohydrates. Percentages that make this diet, much like the Stillman diet, not meet the recommended dietary guidelines that are federally set. Like most of the high-protein diets, Atkins also restricts the consumption of bread, pasta, and starchy vegetables. Potatoes, peas, and corn, is also restricted while alcohol must also be avoided.

Meat, fish, poultry and eggs, butter and oil, and cheese are allowed on this diet. The Atkins diet is, by far, not the safest high-protein diet currently on the market because of its high fat content and should be followed with great caution due to the diet potentially unhealthy on the heart. Health related risks associated with this diet include, colon cancer, and kidney damage. It can also cause bone loss and a condition called ketoacidosis which can cause dieters to feel dizzy, weak, and irritable.

CHAPTER 4- HOW DOES THE PROTEIN DIET FACILITATE WEIGHT LOSS?

One of the most popular diets that have been around for years due to its success is the protein diet. This diet comes in many variations but all of them urge you to increase the amount of protein that you consume each day. Some variations will also recommend decreasing the amount of carbohydrates you consume, in some cases drastically. The protein diet is popular among all groups of people and here are some of the reasons that it facilitates weight loss.

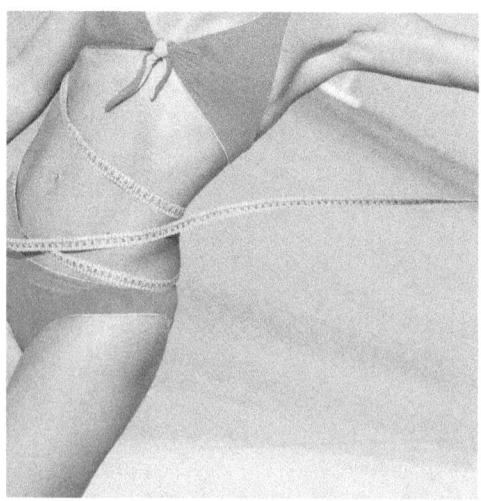

It Works

Before getting into why it works, it is important to understand that increasing the amount of protein you consume does in fact help lose weight or maintain your goal weight. Many people have heard of this and choose to increase their protein consumption to eat more protein. Here is just some of the research supporting the protein diet:

- One study by John Hopkins University found that people who had around 25% of their calories from protein experienced weight loss, lower blood pressure and better cholesterol levels.
- Another study showed that having 30% of your diet come from protein could reduce your daily calorie intake by about 450 amounting to 11 pounds of weight loss.
- A study published by the American Journal of Clinical Nutrition found that a diet of 30% protein led to weight loss, probably due to being less hungry and feeling more satisfied.
- Another study from the University of Illinois showed that eating more protein and fewer carbohydrates can help with weight loss as well as cardiovascular health.

Keeps You Full

One of the reasons that protein is such an effective weight loss tool is that it helps you stay full over time. That is because when you eat foods rich in protein, they will take longer for your body to digest as well as metabolize and use. Because the food remains in your digestive system for longer, you will feel full for a greater period of time. This means that you are less likely to snack. You will even start to feel satisfied earlier on during your meal, encouraging you to eat less.

Some experts think that protein helps reduce your appetite because one of the common proteins triggers something in your brain. They believe this trigger lowers the amount of appetite-stimulating hormones that are released. It also helps that when you eat more protein and fewer carbs or fats you will experience fewer insulin spikes. When there are fewer insulin spikes, your sugar levels won't fluctuate as much, greatly reducing your cravings throughout the day.

Losing Water Weight

Another great benefit of the protein diet is that it helps you lose water weight. It can do this both due to your increased consumption of protein as well as your decreased consumption of carbohydrates. When you include more protein in your diet your amount of albumin (a crucial blood protein) will increase.

This protein is responsible for removing water from your connective tissues and by doing so can reduce fluid retention, helping you lose water weight. One important thing to keep in mind, however, is that because some of the weight you lose on the protein diet is water weight, you may see a slight increase in your weight once you stop the diet.

Fewer Calories

As mentioned earlier, eating more protein helps you stay feel satisfied quicker and stay full for longer which means you will eat less at meals and have fewer snacks, greatly reducing your daily caloric intake. In addition to cutting calories in this way, the versions of the protein diet that reduce carbohydrates can help further reduce calories. That is because many people who are trying to eliminate carbs will simply avoid eating them instead of replacing them. This means that instead of replacing their bread with vegetables, they will simply skip the bread, reducing their calorie count for that meal.

Burns More Calories

We already mentioned that digesting foods rich in protein takes longer than digesting other foods. In addition to helping you stay full for longer, this also means that you burn more calories during the digestion process than you would with other foods. Therefore one of the easiest ways to slightly increase the amount of calories you burn in a day is to opt for protein rich foods and your body will do the rest.

Amino Acids

Because protein is made up amino acids the foods that you eat on the protein diet tend to be rich in multiple different amino acids. Leucine is one of the most important of these amino acids as it can improve your metabolism and therefore weight loss. If you want to make sure that your sources of protein include leucine then you can try the following foods:

- Whey protein
- Cottage cheese
- Red meat
- Milk
- Eggs
- Cheese
- Fish
- Chicken
- Pork
- Seeds
- Nuts
- Peanuts
- Legumes

In addition to helping you lose weight in general, the amino acid leucine is essential at ensuring that you lose fat not muscle when on a diet. If you don't consume enough leucine, your body will lose fat from everywhere and that includes both fat and muscle. When you do consume it, however, it signals the muscles and helps prevent their deterioration.

Helps the Liver with Metabolic Function

Most people who have a basic understanding of biology know that the liver is essential when it comes to your metabolism. What they don't realize is that the protein diet can improve your liver's performance.

When you have a breakfast that contains a great deal of protein your metabolic rate might increase by up to 30 percent and this chance can last for half the day, 12 hours. This is because the liver has to work hard in order to take the proteins apart and then reassemble them so your body can use them in other places. For some comparison, a breakfast that is heavy on carbohydrates and fats will only increase your liver metabolism by 4 percent and that is because they are much easier for it to digest.

CHAPTER 5- 10 PROTEIN DIET BREAKFAST RECIPES

Fried Egg, Italian Sausage with Bacon Sandwich

Ingredients

2 eggs
8 ounces oil
4 small breakfast sausage links
1 slice cheese
1 bagel

Directions

Cut the bacon into tiny cube sizes. Put the 8oz of oil into a frying pan and let it sit on the stove on medium heat for 5 - 7 minutes.

Put the eggs into the frying pan, it should sizzle and turn brown on the bottom side, in 10 seconds flip it over and alternate.

Remove the eggs once they are golden brown, be careful not to burn the inside, only the exterior of the eggs should be slightly golden brown.

Jerk Veggie Burger

Ingredients

2 cans black eyed peas
2 eggs
1 tbsp jerk seasoning
⅓ cup flour
⅓ cup breadcrumbs

Directions

In a small sized bowl mash the 2 cans of black eyed peas until pasty.

Mix the eggs with the black eyed peas.

Add the tablespoon of jerk seasoning into the mixture. Lightly dab the mixture in the flour, and then roll it in the breadcrumbs until it holds together.

You can cook this via grill, frying pan with 1/4 stick of butter or 2 ounces of oil medium heat or the oven at 350 degrees Fahrenheit.

Hot Soy Milk with Almonds Cereal

Ingredients

16 ounce silk (soy milk)
½ cup almonds
1 bowl special k protein cereal

Directions

Cut the almond into small pieces. Mix it into the soy milk.

Microwave the cup of soymilk until hot. Pour it into the bowl of special k protein cereal and let it dissolve. Mix it with 2-3 tablespoons of sugar

Tuna Wrap

Ingredients

2 cans tuna - 5 ounces
1 slice cheese
1 burrito wrap
Mayonnaise
2 slice tomatoes

Directions

Microwave the 4 slices of bacon until desired crisp. Mix the 2 cans of tuna with the mayonnaise in a medium size bowl.

Put it inside the microwave for 1 minute. Mix 1/3 of the stick of butter into the tuna mix and microwave it again for 1 minute.

Serve on the burrito wrap with the slices of cheese, tomatoes and bacon.

Italian Sausage Grinder

Ingredients

1lb Italian sausage
1 6 inch bread roll
2 slices cheese
2 slices tomato

Directions

Cut the sausages midway down forming 'bacon-like' slices.

Put them on the frying pan on medium heat with the 1/3 stick of butter.

Add it to the 6 inch bread roll with the slices of cheese and tomatoes

Veggie Burger

Ingredients

1lb Tofu
Chicken or beef marinade
4oz oil

Cut 1 lb of tofu into 2 slices and place them in a medium sized bowl. Pour the beef or chicken marinade over the two slices of tofu, ensuring you cover them entirely.

Put the container in the freezer and leave it for 24 hrs, this is because tofu will have more of a beef like texture if left frozen overnight.

Thaw the tofu marinade and take those slices out and put them in a separate bowl. Mix and mash the bread crumbs with the tofu along with some sazon seasoning and chicken or beef seasoning.

Mold the mixture into two patties. Heat up the 4oz of oil in a frying pan and place in the pan.

You will be able to tell when the tofu is ready by placing your fork through it; it should feel the same as a beef burger patty would feel when it's done.

Grilled Peanut Butter Jelly Sandwich with Peanut Punch

Florence Perkins
Ingredients

4 slices bread
6 tbsp peanut butter
4 tbsp grape jam
16oz peanut punch

Put 4 tablespoons of peanut butter around the edge but leave the center empty, on one slice of bread, then put 3 tablespoons of jelly in that middle center.

Repeat the same for another slice of bread then cover it. You can grease up an indoor grill and turn the sandwiches until they are crispy brown. Enjoy with some ice cold peanut punch.

Greek Yogurt Banana Cereal

Ingredients

2 cups Greek yogurt
1 bowl raisin bran
1 peach
1 banana

Directions

Cut the peach into 8 slices and cut those into 8 smaller slices. Cut the banana up into 9 slices.

Mix the banana, peach slices in a bowl with the 2 cups of Greek yogurt.

Pour the 8oz of milk into the Greek yogurt mixture and mix it until it's more watery. Pour the mixture into a bowl of raisin bran cereal.

Apple Walnut Oatmeal

Ingredients

1cup oatmeal
1 apple
⅓ cup walnut
3 tbsp sugar
1 tsp cinnamon
½ nutmeg
8oz soy milk

Microwave the soy milk for 1-2 minutes. Pour the oatmeal in the soy milk.

Put the 12 nutmeg in the mixture along with 1 teaspoon of cinnamon, ⅓ cup of walnut and 3 tablespoons of sugar. Mix and microwave the mixture for another 1-2 minutes.

Cut the apple into 16 slices and put it on the oatmeal.

Corned Beef Potato Hash with Eggs

Ingredients

1 can corn beef hash
2 eggs
1 tsp black pepper
Salt
½ onion
⅓ stick of butter

Directions

Put the 1/3 stick of butter in a frying pan on the low heat setting. Cut the onion into small slices and place them in the pan.

Pour 1 teaspoon of black pepper in the pan and mix it around with the onions. Open the can of corn beef hash and put it in the frying pan.

Constantly mix it until its crisp. Take out the corn beef hash, leaving only a few small amounts 'tablespoons worth'.

Put another 1/3 stick of butter with the trace amounts in the pot and stir. Cook the two eggs in the mixture; this will give the eggs a corn beefy flavor itself.

CHAPTER 6- 10 PROTEIN DIET LUNCH RECIPES

Healthy Egg and Spinach Sandwich

Ingredients

Two (2) Cage-Free Large Eggs
Kosher salt
One (1) cup of organic spinach
Two Slices of wheat bread / your choice

Directions

Hard boil your eggs first and set them aside to cool in a refrigerator overnight. The morning of your lunch, steam your spinach and once cooked, season it with kosher salt to your taste, keep this with the eggs until lunch time. To complete for lunch, peel the two hardboiled eggs and slice them 1/4" thick, cover one of the pieces of bread with the egg slices, layer the steamed spinach on top and add the final piece of bread. This sandwich is best served cool.

Pom Cottage Cup

Ingredients

⅔ cup Cottage Cheese
½ cup Pomegranate Seeds

Directions

Obtain your favorite style of cottage cheese with the appropriate fat content that you desire, note that the fat content variation may change the protein content of the meal. Spoon ⅔ of a cup of the chilled cottage cheese into a bowl, then add the pomegranate seeds directly into the cottage cheese and mix. Pomegranate seeds are sometimes sold on their own or a person can harvest them from a pomegranate fruit. Lightly mix the two ingredients to keep texture intact.

Nut House

Ingredients

Bulk Almonds
Bulk Brazil Nuts
Bulk Cashews
Bulk peanuts

Directions

Go to a bulk grocery store or place that sells bulk food and buy 1/4 - 1 lb bags of these nuts, you can choose to buy others if you desire a specific nut. Mix a pre-portioned bag the morning of and bring with you for Lunch. Save what's left over at home for snacks or for lunch on another day.

Tasty Vegan Roll Up

Ingredients

2-3 slices of Tofu turkey (or other low sodium meat substitute)
1 (one) tbsp of Vegan Mayo
1 (one) Slice of Soy Cheese
1 (one) flour tortilla (optional for those who are being carb conscious)

Directions

Layer the "cheese" and "meat" together, roll up loosely as is or with a tortilla to better contain the other ingredients. For an added bonus in the winter time these ingredients can be heated with or without tortilla (careful not to put the cheese on bottom) for 20 seconds in a microwave or 30 seconds over medium heat on a gas range (heat before rolling).

New Style Lentils

Ingredients

1 (one) lb bag of dry lentils
1 (one) tbsp kosher salt
1 (one) tsp cracked black pepper
1 (one) tsp Curry Powder
5 Flax Seed Crackers

Directions

Boil the one pound of lentils in water for 5 minutes the night before they will be cooked, let them simmer for 10 minutes after boiling. Once lentils become thick and cooked thoroughly, add kosher salt, crack black pepper and curry powder directly to cooked lentils. Portion out one cup at a time for consumption, reheat when necessary (refrigerate any leftovers) and eat with flax seed crackers for extra protein. Opt for low sodium crackers as there is already sodium in the lentils from the Kosher Salt.

Apple Oatmeal Crunch

Ingredients

1 (one) cup of Dry Oatmeal
1 (one) Apple (any kind you like)
¼ cup dry banana chips

½ cup water

Directions

Begin with the dry oatmeal oats in a large cup or small bowl the morning you intend on have this meal as your lunch. Slice the apple into 1/4" cubes (or smaller if you prefer). Add the apple to the dry oats and then add the water to this mixture and let the oatmeal soak at room temperature from breakfast until lunch (4-6 hours). Once you are ready for lunch, add your banana chips to the mix.

Almond Paradise

Ingredients

2 (two) Brown Rice Cakes
4 (four) tbsp Almond Butter
2 (two) Organic Strawberries

Directions

Carefully spread almond butter on both rice cakes, minding that the cakes break easily. Slice strawberries and add on top of each cake. Enjoy the cakes one at a time as they will not stack well. Replace Strawberries with other fruit if so desired.

Super Strength Smoothie

Ingredients

1 (one) cup plain Almond Milk
¼ cup frozen Blueberries
¼ cup frozen Mango cubes
¼ cup shredded Kale
½ of a Banana

Directions

Add Blueberries, Mango cubes, Kale (be sure to shred it from the stalk first), and Banana to a blender of your choice. Pour the almond milk over the mix and blend in 20 second intervals until the mix has become liquid enough to drink. The frozen fruit will keep the smoothie cool for longer than unfrozen fruit.

Hemp Seed Peanut Butter

Ingredients

2 tbsp Hemp Seed
1/3 cup Peanut Butter
2 large Celery sticks

Directions

Mix peanut butter with hemp seeds in small container. Spoon out mixture with celery sticks and eat the celery sticks as well!

Hummus Nachos

Ingredients

⅓ cup Hummus
½ a Lemon
10 unsalted Tortilla Chips
¼ cup Soy Cheese Shreds

Directions

Spread the hummus onto one tortilla chip at a time being careful not to break the chips. Squeeze the lemon over the hummus for extra flavor. Add the "cheese" shreds last and heat if prefer them warm.

CHAPTER 7- 10 PROTEIN DIET DINNER RECIPES

The best proteins for any diet are fresh fruits and vegetables, whole grains, leans meats, fish, and poultry. Don't forget to add beans, nuts, eggs, cheese, low fat dairy products and healthy fats. Eat yogurt, fruit, and low fat cheese as a snack instead of a donut or pastry. A protein diet should have about 30 food of the food coming from protein.

Spicy Grilled Chicken Breasts

Ingredients

1 tsp garlic powder
1 tsp chili powder
1 tsp cumin
½ teaspoon crushed red pepper flakes
½ teaspoon salt
2 pounds boneless skinless chicken breast

Directions

With measuring spoon measure spices into a medium sized bowl to use as a rub.

Put chicken breast on a platter rub spices into the chicken breasts on both sides evenly. Put in refrigerator for about 1 hour before grilling.

Grill chicken over medium heat about 10 minutes on each side. Or cook under broiler for about 10 to 15 minutes per side on a baking sheet with foil. Don't forget to spray the sheet or oil grill rack. Serve with steamed vegetables.

Italian Chicken Breasts with Olives

Ingredients

1 can diced tomatoes with Italian spices

1 tablespoon olive oil

½ cup black pitted olives

½ cup green olives pitted

4 small boneless chicken breast about 5 ounces

Directions

Combine canned tomatoes and olives in a bowl. Put aside. In a medium skillet heat oil over medium heat on stove and then add chicken breast and cook about 5 minutes on one side.

Turn the breast over and add tomato olive mixture. Turn down slightly and cook another 5 minutes to 8 minutes or more until chicken is cooked. Serve with noodles or rice.

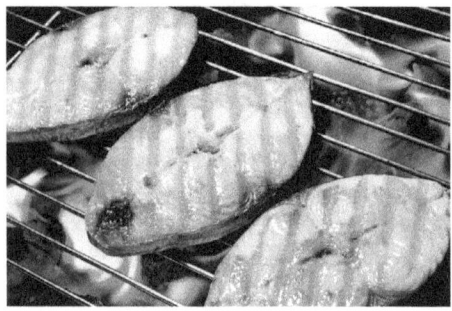

Lemon Pepper Tuna Steaks

Ingredients

½ tsp salt

2 tbsp coarse black pepper

1 tbsp olive oil

1 tbsp lemon juice

Florence Perkins
4 6 ounce tuna steaks

Directions

Combine the spices, oil, and lemon juice in a small bowl. Put the tuna steaks on large platter and rub mixture evenly into both sides.

Put in refrigerator for an hour before grilling. Heat grill or broiler to medium high. Grill tuna steaks about 5 to ten minute per side until done. Serve with steamed vegetables.

Tuna Steaks with Sautéed Red Peppers

Ingredients

2 red bell peppers diced
2 tbsp olive oil
1 tbsp minced garlic
2 five to six ounce tuna steaks
Salt and pepper to taste

Directions

Cut peppers remove seeds and discard. Heat 1 tablespoon oil in frying pan over medium heat and then add garlic and peppers. Cook about 10 to 12 minutes until well cooked. Remove and put peppers in bowl.

On baking sheet with foil put tuna steaks. Spray foil to keep from sticking. Broil tuna steaks about 5 minutes on each side until cooked. Serve on plates with peppers on top of tuna steaks. A salad or brown rice makes a good side dish.

Egg Salad with Basil

Ingredients

4 large white eggs
2 tbsp plain yogurt
1 tsp Dijon mustard
1 tbsp mayonnaise
½ cup washed torn basil leaves
Salt and Pepper to taste

Directions

In a medium sauce pan add cold water and the eggs. Bring to a boil and put lid on it. When it boils turn off pot and let eggs sit in hot water for 10 minutes. Remove from eggs the pan and peel off shell and discard. Chop eggs on cutting board and put in bowl.

Tear or cut basil leaves and add to chopped egg salad. Add plain yogurt, Dijon mustard, and mayonnaise and mix well. Add salt and pepper to taste. Serve on rye or pumpernickel bread as a sandwich or serve as a salad.

Tangy Salmon Salad

Ingredients

1 can of salmon drained
¼ cup minced scallions
2 tomatoes (diced)
1 pickling cucumber peeled, sliced, and quartered
1 tbsp olive oil
1 tbsp lemon juice
Salt and pepper to taste

Directions

Open can of salmon and drain off juice. Add to the medium sized bowl. On cutting board chop scallions and add to salmons mix well with fork.

Wash and dice tomatoes add to salad. Peel and dice small cucumbers add to bowl. Add oil and lemon juice toss well. Add salt and pepper. Serve as a salad or on whole wheat bread as a sandwich.

Tomato and Cheddar Cheese Sandwiches

Ingredients

2 large tomatoes washed and sliced thin
¼ pound cheddar cheese sliced thin
Slices of whole wheat bread
1 tbsp olive oil
¼ tsp chopped garlic
¼ tsp basil
Salt and pepper to taste

Directions

Wash and cut the tomatoes into thin slices. Put on plate. Arrange the bread and lay two slices of cheddar cheese on each slice of bread. Top with two slices of tomato.

Mix the olive oil, chopped garlic, and basil in small bowl. Drizzle on top of tomatoes. Add other slice of bread and cut sandwiches in half. Serve with a salad.

Spicy Grilled Rib Eye Steak Recipes

Ingredients

1 tsp chili powder
¼ tsp cayenne pepper
1 tsp garlic powder
1 tsp black pepper
2 lbs of rib eye steaks

Directions

In a bowl mix all the dry spice ingredients. Put the steaks on a flat platter and plate.

Rub the spice mixture evenly into both sides of the steak. Let sit in refrigerator about 1 hour.

Oil the grill and heat to medium heat or grill under broiler. Grill steaks on both sides about 10 minutes each side until done. Serve with steamed vegetables and a salad.

Spicy Flank Steak with Chili Lime Marinade

¼ cup lime juice
2 tbsp chili powder
1 tbsp olive oil
1 tbsp dark soy sauce
Salt and pepper to taste
2 pounds flank steak

Directions

Mix the lime juice, chili powder, olive oil, and dark soy sauce in bowl. Mix well. Put the flank steak in a Ziploc bag and add marinade. Leave in refrigerator at least 2 to 4 hours.

Heat grill to high and oil and place steak on it. If using a broiler use baking sheet with foil sprayed with vegetable oil. Cook about 8 to 10 minutes on each side. Let rest and slice thinly. Serve with brown rice.

ABOUT THE AUTHOR

Florence Perkins grew up in a family that was strictly vegan but when she became an adult she became interested in trying new things without making the wrong choices which would end up with her gaining unnecessary weight. She made the decision to play it safe and ended up choosing the protein diet as something to try. She would get to try a variety of meats without worrying that she would get fat.

She had the blessing of her family as though they chose to be vegan; they had no objections to their children trying new things. Florence found the diet to be quite tasty and extremely beneficial. She was able to maintain her weight as well. As a result of this she became a supporter of the diet to the point where she ended up writing her own book about it.

www.ingramcontent.com/pod-product-compliance
Lightning Source LLC
Chambersburg PA
CBHW060344290526
45791CB00004B/1522